Revitalize Your Life

7 Transformative Tips for Busy Women Reclaiming Wellness

JODY DOTSON

Revitalize Your Life

Contact: JodyDHealthCoach.com
jody@jodydotson.com

ISBN: 978-1-7342323-6-3
Printed in the United States of America

Book cover design and Interior formatting by 100 Covers.

DEDICATION

This book is lovingly dedicated to the incredible women who are the true architects of their lives, tirelessly navigating the intricate tapestry of responsibilities and aspirations. To every busy woman out there who feels like she's chasing after elusive extra hours in the day – this one's for you. Whether you're a powerhouse career woman, a devoted mother, a compassionate caregiver, or a fearless entrepreneur or CEO, this dedication is a heartfelt acknowledgment of the challenges you face and the triumphs you achieve on a daily basis.

I want to express my deepest admiration and respect for the way you take on the world, wearing multiple hats and gracefully managing the delicate balance between personal and professional spheres. It's not lost on me that you might sometimes feel like a magician trying to pull an extra hour out of thin air, desperately seeking a pause button in the chaotic rhythm of life.

To the career women boldly making strides in their chosen fields – your ambition and dedication are awe-inspiring. To the mothers pouring love into every hug, kiss, and scraped knee – your nurturing spirit shapes the future. To the caregivers providing comfort and support to those in need – your selflessness is a beacon of compassion. And to the entrepreneurs and CEOs shaping industries and driving innovation – your vision and leadership propel us forward.

This dedication is more than just words; it's a promise. A promise that you don't have to sacrifice your health and wellness at the altar of success. Within these pages, I share not only insights and wisdom but also a genuine belief that a healthy, happy, and balanced life is not an unattainable myth. It's a reality waiting to be embraced, and you deserve to revel in it.

As you embark on this journey through the chapters ahead, envision it as a companion whispering in your ear, cheering you on, and reminding you that self-care is not a luxury; it's a necessity. Here's to finding joy in the everyday moments, to embracing a slower pace when needed, and to understanding that your well-being is an integral part of your success story.

Thank you for being the extraordinary woman that you are – resilient, determined, and capable of rewriting the narrative. May this book be a source of inspiration, guidance, and a gentle nudge to prioritize your health and happiness, because you deserve nothing less.

CONTENTS

INTRODUCTION

A few years ago, I found myself struggling with my health. Perhaps you can relate. Have you ever felt like no matter how much you exercise or diet, you can't seem to shed those last few pounds? Or maybe you've experienced that midday slump after indulging in multiple Mocha Frappuccinos, feeling drained and sluggish as the day progresses. I can assure you that I have been there.

Not long ago, I was caught in a cycle of trying various diets, investing in exercise programs, and even hiring personal trainers to improve my health. However, despite my efforts, I couldn't achieve *my* desired results. It was frustrating and disheartening. It wasn't until I took a step back and examined the root cause of my struggles that I could make a breakthrough.

I discovered that stress, low energy levels, and a general feeling of unfulfillment were at the core of my health issues. Recognizing this made me understand that focusing on diet and exercise was not enough. I needed to address these underlying factors to achieve true and lasting change.

This realization sparked a transformation within me. I became passionate about understanding the intricate connections between physical and mental well-being. I delved into the world of nutrition, lifestyle medicine, and holistic approaches to health. Through my journey, I discovered the incredible healing power within our bodies, given the right tools and support.

Motivated by my personal experience, I embarked on a new path as a health and wellness coach. My mission was clear – to guide and empower others on their transformative journeys. I firmly believe that our bodies have an innate ability to heal themselves. We can enhance this healing process by embracing lifestyle medicine and reclaiming our health.

Today, as a health coach, I specialize in helping busy working women transform their lives. I work closely with my clients to help them shed excess weight, adopt healthier eating habits, and regain energy. My ultimate goal is to empower them to feel confident and in control of their health and well-being.

Throughout this book, I will share the knowledge, strategies, and practical advice I have acquired over the years. I will provide the tools you need to embark on your journey toward better health. I sincerely hope this book serves as a guiding light, illuminating the path toward a healthier, happier, and more fulfilling life.

The chapters within this book unravel conventional notions of health and guide you toward a more sustainable and meaningful path. In these pages, you'll discover that the pursuit of wellness transcends rigid diets and quick fixes. From ditching traditional diets that promise miracles to embracing a holistic approach that nourishes your body, mind, and soul, you'll learn to craft a wellness journey that is uniquely your own.

The chapters delve into a mosaic of topics, each shedding light on a different holistic and nutritional wellness facet. From understanding the profound impact of stress and the art of energy restoration to navigating the intricacies of workplace nutrition and the transformative power of removing sugar from your daily diet, you'll find practical insights and actionable steps to enhance your well-being. Moreover, this book explores the potential for nutrition and lifestyle practices to reverse chronic illness, proving that wellness is an ongoing journey that can yield life-changing results.

You'll also encounter the art of self-care, a cornerstone of holistic wellness. In a world that often glorifies busyness, the chapters emphasize the importance of nurturing yourself, setting boundaries, and fostering connections that uplift your spirit. Each chapter is a step forward in your well-being.

I work with many women to assist them with their weight loss and wellness journeys. I remember working with a client named Allison, who struggled with her weight and self-image after giving birth to her second child. Together, we developed a personalized plan that included a balanced meal plan focused on clean eating. I educated Allison on the significance of whole foods, portion control, and mindful eating. We also integrated regular exercise into her routine, based on her preferences and schedule, to make it enjoyable and maintainable. As weeks passed, Allison's dedication and commitment started yielding remarkable results. She lost an incredible 42 pounds, and more importantly, she experienced a renewed sense of self-esteem and confidence. By adopting a clean eating lifestyle, Allison not only shed weight but also noticed improvements in her energy levels and overall well-being. She discovered a passion for nutritious foods and realized that caring for her body was a form of self-love.

I had another client, Lisa, who was determined to break free from her sugar addiction and embrace a healthier lifestyle. She took the first step by purchasing my 10-day sugar detox program, seeking guidance and structure to kickstart her journey. During the 10-day program, Lisa showed remarkable commitment and willpower. She diligently followed the program, eliminating sugary foods and beverages from her regimen. As a result, she experienced a significant reduction in cravings and noticed positive changes in her energy levels, which inspired Lisa to take her health journey further. Lisa sought out my continued ongoing support. Throughout our coaching sessions, we delved deeper into the emotional aspects of her sugar cravings, exploring the triggers behind them. I provided tools and strategies to cope with stress and emotions in healthier ways, helping her build a strong foundation for sustainable changes. As the weeks passed, Lisa continuously resisted sugary temptations and incorporated more nutritious eating habits into her daily life. She experienced gradual weight loss, further motivating her to stay on track. We also explored various aspects of well-being, including exercise, sleep, and self-care. Lisa's enthusiasm grew, and she embraced a more holistic approach to her health. By the end of the coaching program, Lisa had not only conquered her sugar addiction but had also developed a positive relationship with food and her body. She felt empowered, confident, and ready to maintain her newfound healthy lifestyle.

Like Allison, Lisa, and many more, I want you to experience success in living a healthier, well-balanced life. This journey is not about perfection; it's about intention. It's about embracing your uniqueness, nurturing your health, and honoring the journey toward holistic and nutritional wellness with patience, self-compassion, and a deep sense of purpose. The following chapters will guide you on this journey, offering insights, strategies, and inspiration to help you create a life that radiates well-being in every facet. Your wellness story is as unique as you are, and this book is a compass to help you navigate the path toward a healthier, more vibrant, and empowered life.

As a thank you for reading this book, I would like to offer you a free gift, *3 Ways To Quit Sugar When You'd Kill For A Cookie*. To access your copy, visit this link: https://pages.jodydhealthcoach.com/sugar.

CHAPTER 1

Breaking Free
Liberating Yourself from the Dieting Trap

"The food you eat can be either the safest and most powerful form of medicine or the slowest form of poison."
– Ann Wigmore

In a world consumed by quick fixes and ever-changing beauty standards, the allure of diets often takes center stage. The concept of a diet, a temporary and often restrictive eating regimen designed to achieve specific goals, has been ingrained in our culture as a means to attain the coveted ideal body. Yet, beneath the surface of these well-marketed solutions lies a truth many have realized: diets don't work. Pursuing instant results through deprivation and rigid rules seldom leads to lasting health or contentment. This chapter embarks on a journey of liberation from the cycle of diets, aiming to reframe how women approach nutrition and well-being.

While seemingly promising, diets ultimately fall short of delivering the transformative changes they advertise. The reasons are manifold, ranging from their inherently unsustainable nature to the physiological and psychological toll they impose. Restrictive eating patterns disrupt the body's natural equilibrium, often leading to rebound weight gain once the diet ends. The strictures they place on food can foster guilt, shame, and an unhealthy relationship with nourishment. Moreover, diets tend to focus solely on the physical aspect of health, overlooking the integral roles that mental and emotional well-being play in achieving holistic vitality. A profound understanding emerges as the curtain is pulled back on the illusions diets cast: the path to genuine wellness requires a departure from this cycle.

Recognizing the shortcomings of diets lays the foundation for a paradigm shift towards a healthier and more sustainable approach to nutrition. Beyond the confines of rigid meal plans and quick fixes lies a realm where balanced nourishment and overall well-being are the focal points. The call to embrace a holistic perspective takes root as women begin to understand that their bodies deserve respect, nourishment, and care. It's a shift from external ideals to intrinsic empowerment, from chasing numbers on a scale to cultivating energy, vitality, and a positive self-image. This chapter embarks on a journey that will encourage you to step away from diets and embark on a path that prioritizes sustainable health, self-compassion, and a newfound appreciation for the beauty of balanced well-being.

Understanding the Diet Mindset

Within the intricate landscape of our modern lives, the diet mentality emerges as a formidable force that can shape our perceptions of self and well-being. The diet mindset, rooted in pursuing an elusive ideal, promises transformation through restriction and discipline. However, beneath its surface allure lies a treacherous path laden with harmful behaviors and distorted self-images. The diet mentality fosters a relentless pursuit of perfection, often leading individuals to view food as a source of guilt and self-punishment. This mindset's gravitational pull toward unrealistic body standards can cultivate feelings of inadequacy and perpetuate a cycle of negativity that sabotages not only physical health but also mental well-being.

Inextricably intertwined with the diet mentality is the pervasive influence of diet culture. A formidable presence in media, advertising, and even interpersonal interactions, diet culture significantly impacts how we perceive our bodies and our relationship with food. It promotes the notion that worthiness is contingent upon adherence to specific beauty standards and food choices. The result is a fractured connection with our bodies, fostering shame and discontent. Our once harmonious relationship with food becomes fraught with anxiety and over-analysis, leading to disordered eating patterns. The constant barrage of messages championing rapid fixes further fuels this tumultuous cycle, often obscuring the deeper understanding that genuine health extends beyond numbers on a scale.

At the heart of the diet mindset lies the cycle of restrictive eating, a pattern that often ensnares individuals in a web of physical and psychological consequences. Initially publicized as a means of control and transformation, restrictive eating can rapidly deteriorate into an all-consuming obsession. The irony lies in its contradictory nature: the more one attempts to control and restrict, the more the body and mind resist. This rebellion often results in binge-eating episodes, followed by intense guilt and shame. The cycle perpetuates a sense of powerlessness, eroding self-esteem and amplifying negative self-talk. Over time, the physical toll of such erratic eating patterns becomes evident, disrupting metabolism, hormonal balance, and overall vitality. Simultaneously, the mental toll can lead to anxiety, depression, and a pervasive sense of failure. By unraveling this cycle, we can reconstruct a healthier relationship with food, our bodies, and ourselves, embracing a path that prioritizes nourishment, self-compassion, and holistic well-being.

In the realm of the diet mindset, the interplay of perceptions, culture, and behaviors is a complex dance that shapes our approach to health and self. Understanding its intricacies is the first step toward dismantling its grip, fostering a renewed connection with our bodies and nourishment that transcends the limitations of traditional dieting.

Understanding Diets

Our relationship with diets is intertwined often with societal pressures and cultural expectations. Common characteristics of diets aimed at women frequently include promises of rapid weight loss, often driven by restrictive eating patterns or elimination of entire food groups. While these diets might yield initial results, they pose significant risks. The cycle of weight loss and regain can disrupt metabolism, leading to a potential long-term struggle with weight fluctuations and even eating disorders. The pursuit of thinness can also foster negative body image and feelings of inadequacy, impacting not only physical health but emotional well-being. Acknowledging these risks is crucial in steering women toward healthier, more sustainable approaches that prioritize overall health and self-acceptance.

The allure of fad diets often lies in their promise of quick fixes and dramatic transformations. However, the distinction between short-term and long-term effects is pivotal. While fad diets might showcase immediate results, they frequently fail to address the broader picture of sustainable health. Rapid weight loss, often from water and muscle loss, can mask the true impact on overall body composition. These diets seldom account for the importance of balanced nutrition, which is pivotal in maintaining energy levels, hormonal balance, and overall vitality. By shifting the focus from immediate outcomes to lasting well-being, you can make informed choices that prioritize your holistic health journey.

The landscape of popular diet trends is loaded with misconceptions that can lead you astray. From demonizing certain macronutrients to promoting extreme calorie deficits, these trends perpetuate a distorted view of nutrition. Keto diets, for instance, may lead to short-term weight loss but often neglect the importance of sustainable carbohydrate intake for brain function and energy. Similarly, detox and cleanse diets can mislead you into thinking you can "reset" your body through short-term deprivation, disregarding the body's innate detoxification mechanisms. By debunking these misconceptions and focusing on evidence-based approaches, you can make empowered choices that prioritize nourishment, balanced eating, and a realistic understanding of your body's needs.

In the intricate realm of dieting, navigating beyond surface-level promises and quick fixes is crucial. By understanding common dieting practices' characteristics, risks, and consequences, women can embrace a journey that prioritizes long-term health, body positivity, and a more nuanced approach to well-being.

Suggested Alternatives

Shifting away from the restrictive confines of diets, you can discover a realm of sustainable health by embracing balanced nutrition. Rather than fixating on caloric restrictions, the emphasis is on nourishing the body with diverse nutrients. Recognizing each nutrient's unique role in our well-being, you can cultivate a dietary pattern that promotes energy, vitality, and optimal functioning. By viewing food as fuel for body and mind, the focus expands beyond weight and appearance to encompass the broader wellness spectrum.

A cornerstone of fostering optimal health lies in constructing a foundation of nutrient-dense foods. This approach centers on incorporating whole, minimally processed foods that provide a rich spectrum of vitamins, minerals, and antioxidants. Colorful vegetables, lean proteins, whole grains, and healthy fats become the building blocks of nourishment. Beyond immediate physical benefits, nutrient-dense choices contribute to long-term well-being by supporting immune function, hormonal balance, and even mental clarity. You can harness the power of these foods to empower your body, fortifying yourself against the pitfalls of restrictive dieting.

Mindful eating emerges as a powerful alternative to the cycles of guilt and restriction. It encourages you to listen to your body's cues, honoring hunger and fullness signals without judgment. By savoring each bite and cultivating a conscious connection with the act of eating, you can reframe your relationship with food. This approach frees them from the emotional roller coaster often associated with dieting, fostering a friendly rapport with nourishment. Coupled with this, cultivating a positive and healthy relationship with food involves shedding the labels of "good" and "bad" and embracing the idea that all foods have a place in a balanced diet. By removing the stigma surrounding certain foods, you can find joy in eating without the weight of guilt or restriction.

As you embark on a journey beyond diets, you unveil a realm of nourishment that transcends fleeting transformations. By prioritizing balanced nutrition, embracing nutrient-dense choices, practicing mindful eating, and fostering a positive relationship with food, you can forge a path that celebrates your body and nurtures your holistic well-being.

Sustainable Lifestyle Changes

In pursuit of sustainable well-being, you can pivot from the narrow focus of diets to the expansive realm of movement and exercise. Rather than viewing physical activity as a means to burn calories, it becomes a gateway to improved health and vitality. Engaging in activities that bring joy, like dancing, hiking, or practicing yoga, encourages a lifelong commitment to movement. Regular exercise supports cardiovascular health and muscular strength and nurtures mental well-being by releasing endorphins and reducing stress. By embracing movement as an integral part of your life, you cultivate a harmonious relationship with your body, fostering a sense of empowerment and agency.

Shifting the focus from diets to sustainable lifestyle changes involves weaving a tapestry of healthy routines and supportive habits. Consistent sleep patterns, adequate hydration, and regular meal times lay the foundation for balanced well-being. These routines provide a stable framework that encourages mindful eating and supports overall metabolic health. Integrating a variety of nutrient-rich foods into daily meals offers a steady stream of energy and nourishment. Surrounding oneself with a supportive community further bolsters these efforts, offering encouragement and accountability on the journey toward lasting wellness.

One of the most profound shifts in sustainable wellness involves cultivating emotional resilience and stress management. Replacing the tendency to turn to food or restrictive eating as coping mechanisms, you can explore alternative strategies to navigate stress and emotions. Practices such as meditation, deep breathing, and mindfulness offer tools to respond to stressors with clarity and poise. Building emotional awareness enables you to differentiate between actual hunger and emotional cravings. By embracing healthier outlets for emotional expression, such as journaling, creative endeavors, or seeking support from trusted individuals, you foster a profound connection between emotional well-being and physical health, anchoring yourself in a journey of holistic self-care.

As you embark on the path of sustainable lifestyle changes, you redefine your relationship with health, embracing movement, cultivating routines, and managing emotions in ways that transcend the confines of diets. By weaving these practices into the fabric of your life, you can attain a sense of empowerment, resilience, and lasting well-being that flourishes far beyond the transient nature of restrictive eating approaches.

Summary

In this comprehensive exploration of your well-being, the multifaceted landscape of dieting is unveiled and navigated with a fresh perspective. The chapters dive into the complexities of the diet mindset, shedding light on its harmful effects on self-image and behaviors. They emphasize the detrimental impact of diet culture on our relationship with food and body image, revealing how misconceptions surrounding popular trends can lead women astray. As you traverse this intricate terrain, sustainable alternatives to diets become illuminated, guiding you toward a transformative path.

Action Steps:

1. Mindset Awareness: Reflect on your relationship with diet, diet culture, and body image. Identify moments where the diet mentality has influenced your thoughts and behaviors.
2. Educate Yourself: Research popular diet trends' characteristics, risks, and short-term vs. long-term effects. Seek out evidence-based information to make informed choices.
3. Holistic Habits: Establish a routine that encompasses movement, sleep, hydration, and mindful eating. Engage in physical activity that brings joy and supports your well-being. What will you add to your routine?

Incorporating the wisdom gleaned from understanding the pitfalls of diets, debunking misconceptions, and embracing nourishment, you can embark on a journey that prioritizes holistic well-being over short-lived transformations. By cultivating healthier relationships with food, movement, emotions, and your body, you can sustainably empower yourself, fostering a sense of agency and positivity that transcends the superficial confines of dieting.

CHAPTER 2

Stress Mastery

Strategies for a Balanced Life

"Take care of your body. It's the only place you have to live."
–Jim Rohn

In the fast-paced modern landscape, stress has become an unwelcome companion for many, particularly for the ever-busy working women who often bear the weight of multiple responsibilities. Stress, a natural response to the demands of life, has the power to shape our experiences and influence our well-being in profound ways. For women, the juggling act of work, family, and personal aspirations can manifest as a unique tapestry of stressors. Recognizing the intricate role stress plays in your life is pivotal in unraveling its impact on both your mental and physical realms. This chapter embarks on a journey through the realm of stress mastery and will empower you with tools to navigate life's demands while nurturing your holistic well-being.

For busy working women, stress often takes on a multifaceted form. It might manifest as a relentless sense of urgency, a ceaseless stream of tasks, or a constant tug-of-war between professional and personal commitments. The weight of these responsibilities can seep into your mental and emotional landscapes, causing fatigue, irritability, and an overwhelming feeling of being stretched too thin. Physically, stress can lead to disrupted sleep patterns, tension, and even more severe health issues if left unchecked. As this chapter delves into the labyrinth of stress, a clearer picture emerges of its toll on you, hopefully urging you to seek a path toward mastery.

The impact of stress goes beyond fleeting moments of pressure; it weaves its threads into the fabric of mental and physical health. Mentally, chronic stress can lead to anxiety, mood swings, and an inability to focus, gradually eroding overall cognitive function. Physically, the effects can range from digestive disturbances to weakened immune responses, making individuals more susceptible to illnesses. The intricate interplay between mind and body underscores the need for a comprehensive approach to stress management. This chapter aims to equip you with strategies to mitigate the toll of stress, fostering a sense of empowerment over your mental and physical well-being.

As the demands of modern life continue to evolve, stress mastery emerges as an essential skill for maintaining overall well-being. The ability to manage stress not only bolsters your emotional resilience but also safeguards your physical health. By recognizing stress's presence, understanding its effects, and arming themselves with effective stress management techniques, women can forge a path to greater equilibrium. This chapter sets the stage for a transformative journey, inviting you to navigate life's challenges with grace and poise, embracing the serenity that comes from mastering stress for the betterment of your holistic health.

Recognizing the Signs and Causes of Stress

Stress manifests in various forms that demand our attention. Two prominent types, acute and chronic stress, paint distinct strokes on this canvas. Acute stress, often arising from immediate challenges or deadlines, triggers a temporary surge of adrenaline and heightened awareness. On the other hand, chronic stress weaves a continuous thread, stemming from persistent demands and enduring pressures, and can silently erode our well-being over time. Identifying these types is the first step in understanding how stress manifests in our lives.

Recognizing the more subtle nuances of stress involves understanding its telltale signs and symptoms. These indicators often permeate multiple dimensions of our being. Emotionally, stress might manifest as irritability, anxiety, or a sense of being overwhelmed. Physically, it can evoke tension, headaches, digestive issues, and even disrupted sleep patterns. Cognitive symptoms include difficulty concentrating, forgetfulness, and a constant state of racing thoughts. By being attuned to these signals, we can begin to address stress's impact on our holistic health.

Beneath the surface of these signs lies a labyrinth of causes and triggers unique to each individual's life. Stress can stem from a wide array of sources - from work-related pressures and financial concerns to relationship dynamics and personal aspirations. Exploring the underlying causes involves delving into the complex interplay of external demands and internal responses. Identifying these triggers is vital, as it provides insight into the patterns that perpetuate stress and allows you to craft tailored strategies for effective stress management. By unraveling these threads, you gain agency over your response to stress, paving the way for a more harmonious and resilient existence.

Stress Reduction Techniques

Amid the whirlwind of modern life, stress reduction techniques offer a lifeline to reclaim tranquility and inner balance. Mindfulness, the art of being fully present in the moment, stands as a cornerstone of these practices. Embracing mindfulness fosters an intimate connection with the present, unraveling the threads of anxiety woven by past regrets and future worries. Incorporating mindfulness into your everyday routine can be as simple as dedicating moments to focused breathing or engaging in sensory awareness, grounding you in the present and providing a sanctuary of calm amidst the chaos.

Meditation, an age-old practice, is a potent conduit to cultivate mindfulness. By dedicating time to stillness and turning your attention inward, meditation offers a respite from the demands of external stimuli. Guided meditation sessions, body scan exercises, or mantra repetition can serve as your sanctuary of inner peace. Integrating mindfulness techniques into your daily routine, such as mindful eating, walking, or even brushing your teeth, extends the practice's benefits into your everyday life. This conscious presence grants you a moment of reprieve from the rapid pace of life and a chance to reconnect with yourself.

Navigating the ebb and flow of emotions is a vital facet of stress reduction. Cultivating coping strategies that channel emotions constructively empowers you to navigate life's challenges with grace. Breathing techniques, like the 4-7-8 method, can swiftly shift your body's stress response, offering a calming counterbalance. Utilizing stress-relief apps that offer guided meditation or relaxation exercises extends an accessible means to manage stress anytime, anywhere. Engaging in physical activity, whether it's yoga, running, or dancing, serves as an outlet to release pent-up tension and uplift your spirits. These strategies provide a nurturing space for emotional expression, acting as an essential armor against the daily onslaught of stressors.

Designing a harmonious environment contributes significantly to stress reduction. Decluttering your space fosters clarity of mind and allows for mental space to flourish. Infusing your surroundings with calming elements, such as soothing colors, plants, or natural lighting, sets the stage for relaxation. Engaging the senses through aromatherapy, calming music, or tactile objects enhances sensory experiences, acting as a balm for frayed nerves. Moreover, fostering a work-life balance tailored to support your well-being is pivotal. Establishing boundaries, unplugging digital devices, and scheduling regular breaks all contribute to a balanced rhythm that bolsters stress management.

Integrating mindfulness, meditation, healthy coping strategies, and an optimal environment creates a symphony of practices that orchestrate serenity as you embark on your journey toward stress reduction. These techniques empower you to take charge of your well-being, nurturing resilience, and fostering a sense of agency over life's challenges. By carving out these pockets of tranquility, you weave a tapestry of inner strength that becomes your foundation for navigating the intricate tapestry of modern life with grace and poise.

Summary

Navigating the intricate landscape of stress involves recognizing its various manifestations, from acute to chronic stress, and understanding the subtle signs that permeate our mental, emotional, and physical realms. We gain insight into our unique stressors by acknowledging the underlying causes and triggers that fuel stress. This awareness serves as the foundation for crafting strategies that foster serenity and holistic well-being.

Action Steps:

1. Self-Reflection and Journaling: Dedicate time to reflect on recent experiences that caused stress. Journal your observations of physical, emotional, and cognitive signs of stress. Use this record to identify patterns and recurring triggers.

2. Mindful Breathing Practice: Set aside a few minutes daily for mindful breathing. Close your eyes, take deliberate breaths, and focus on the sensations of inhaling and exhaling. Observe how this practice brings you into the present moment, alleviating stress. Recommended apps: https://www.calm.com and https://balanceapp.com

3. Mindful Moment Integration: Select a routine activity, like eating or showering, to infuse with mindfulness. Engage all your senses during this activity and immerse yourself fully in the experience.

4. Identify a strategy that will be your go-to for managing a stressful situation.

As you navigate stress with increased awareness and integrate mindfulness practices into your routine, you'll find yourself better equipped to manage life's challenges. By cultivating serenity within yourself and your environment, you empower yourself to embrace life with grace, resilience, and a renewed sense of balance.

CHAPTER 3

From Fatigue to Fabulous

Unleashing Your Inner Powerhouse

"What most people don't realize is that food is not just calories; it's information. It actually contains messages that connect to every cell in the body."
– Dr. Mark Hyman

In picturing your overall well-being, there exists a spot that often goes unnoticed: energy. Far beyond the superficial realm of appearances, energy is the life force that underpins productivity, mental clarity, and the overall quality of life. From the moment we awaken until we lay our heads to rest, energy courses through our veins, propelling us forward in our pursuits. This chapter delves into the profound significance of energy well-being, unraveling its impact on productivity, focus, and every facet of our existence. By understanding the sources of energy, the interplay of nutrition, and the power of energy-boosting foods, you can embark on a journey of holistic vitality.

Energy is not merely a fleeting surge but a symphony orchestrating our daily activities. It wields an undeniable influence over our ability to meet deadlines, maintain focus, and engage in meaningful interactions. Just as a lack of energy can cast shadows on our potential, harnessing energy with intention has the power to elevate our well-being to unparalleled heights. The connection between energy and overall health is profound, intertwining the physical, mental, and emotional realms. By embracing energy well-being, you can unlock a source of untapped potential that resonates through every aspect of your life.

To comprehend energy well-being is to understand the multifaceted sources from which energy originates. Beyond the obvious source of sleep, energy is derived from the intricate interplay of nutrition, physical activity, and mental harmony. The foods we consume act as fuel, dictating the vigor with which we approach our days. This chapter delves into the role of nutrition as a cornerstone of energy cultivation, exploring the significance of balanced meals and the impact of energy-boosting foods. By deciphering these sources, you gain insight into the harmonious rhythm that governs your energy levels and, subsequently, your overall wellness.

Fueling the body with energy-boosting foods becomes an empowering act of self-care, allowing women to seize each day with renewed vitality. These foods, rich in nutrients, complex carbohydrates, and essential vitamins, serve as catalysts that sustain energy levels and stave off midday slumps. This chapter navigates through a landscape of energy-boosting foods, unveiling their roles in enhancing alertness, combating fatigue, and promoting mental clarity. By integrating these foods into your diet, you not only experience heightened physical energy but also lay the foundation for balanced well-being that radiates from the inside out.

In the following pages, you will embark on an exploration of energy well-being, peeling back the layers to understand its profound impact on productivity, focus, and quality of life. From the sources of energy to the role of nutrition and the energy-boosting foods that elevate us, this chapter is a roadmap to nurturing vitality at its core. As you grasp the significance of energy well-being, you empower yourself to navigate life's demands with a renewed vigor that transcends the ordinary and blossoms into holistic health.

Understanding the Impacts of Energy

In the bustling world of a busy working woman, energy operates as the invisible force that holds the key to unlocking productivity, enhancing focus, and shaping the overall quality of life. Picture a day that begins with a well-rested night's sleep, infusing the body with revitalizing energy. As tasks unfold, energy becomes the driving force behind productivity, enabling you to tackle challenges with precision and efficacy. With every ounce of energy harnessed, deadlines are met, projects are executed with finesse, and the to-do list dwindles under the influence of your vigor.

Focus, that elusive gem of concentration, is intricately interwoven with energy. When energy levels are optimal, the mind becomes a laser beam of attention, absorbing information, making decisions, and problem-solving with remarkable clarity. A wellspring of energy empowers you to navigate the intricacies of your responsibilities without succumbing to the mental fog that often accompanies fatigue. In these moments, energy is a supportive ally, fortifying your ability to remain fully immersed in your tasks, undistracted by the pull of weariness.

Beyond productivity and focus, energy imparts a transformative touch to the overall quality of your life. Energized days allow for meaningful interactions, where connections are fostered without the burden of exhaustion. Conversations are infused with vitality, laughter, and genuine engagement, enriching both your personal and professional relationships. With abundant energy as your companion, you carve out time for self-care, pursuing hobbies, and cherishing moments that add layers of vibrancy to your existence. In this delicate balance, energy emerges as the cornerstone that elevates the quality of your life, creating a harmonious blend of fulfillment, success, and well-being.

Understanding Energy Sources

Energy sources take center stage as the vital components that power your everyday endeavors. These sources are diverse, spanning the realms of physical, mental, emotional, and even spiritual well-being. At the core of your energy foundation lies physical vitality, fueled by restorative sleep, nourishing nutrition, and regular physical activity. This physical energy equips you to tackle your responsibilities with stamina and vigor.

Mental energy serves as the cognitive engine that powers your thoughts, decision-making, and problem-solving capabilities. Much like a battery, it requires regular replenishment to maintain optimal performance. Meditation, where you consciously direct your focus inward and cultivate mindfulness, acts as a reset button for your mind. This practice allows you to declutter mental clutter, reduce stress, and restore mental clarity. Engaging in brief breaks throughout the day, even for just a few minutes, offers your mind the chance to recalibrate, preventing mental fatigue and boosting overall cognitive efficiency.

Furthermore, hobbies, the pursuits that ignite your passion and creativity, play a pivotal role in recharging your mental energy. Whether it's painting, playing a musical instrument, or indulging in a favorite sport, hobbies provide a sanctuary where your mind can wander freely and detach from work-related stressors. These activities stimulate your brain in novel ways, fostering cognitive flexibility and rejuvenating your mental reserves. As you dedicate time to these hobbies, you not only rejuvenate your mental energy but also tap into a source of joy that enriches your overall well-being.

Emotional energy, often likened to the nourishment that sustains plants, requires dedicated care to flourish. Meaningful relationships, where you share experiences, support, and laughter with loved ones, act as emotional anchors. Just as plants thrive with regular watering, your emotional well-being flourishes when you invest time and effort into fostering these connections. Carving out personal time for yourself is equally vital. Engaging in activities you love, whether reading a book, taking a leisurely walk, or simply unwinding with a warm bath, provides the emotional self-care that prevents burnout and nurtures your emotional equilibrium.

Stress-relief practices, such as deep breathing exercises or journaling, offer outlets for releasing accumulated tension and processing emotions. Just as plants require sunlight to thrive, these practices provide your emotional landscape with the light of self-awareness and emotional release. By embracing these strategies and recognizing the significance of mental and emotional well-being, you craft a fortified inner landscape that equips you to navigate the demands of your busy life with resilience, creativity, and a profound sense of balance.

However, as in any delicate ecosystem, energy is susceptible to depletion. External factors, such as excessive workloads or draining relationships, can siphon away energy. Internal factors, including negative self-talk and unresolved emotions, also play a role in draining your vitality. Recognizing these potential energy drains is a pivotal step in protecting and optimizing your energy sources. By consciously replenishing and safeguarding your energy reserves, you craft a life that resonates with vibrancy, balance, and overall well-being.

Fueling Your Body Through Nutrition

Nutrition serves as the cornerstone of energy well-being, offering the body the fuel it requires to power through the demands of your life. Like a well-tuned engine, the body thrives when nourished with a balanced combination of nutrients. Carbohydrates, the body's primary energy source, provide the immediate burst of energy needed to kickstart the day. Complex carbohydrates found in whole grains, fruits, and vegetables release energy steadily, preventing energy crashes and providing sustained vitality. Pairing these with lean proteins, such as poultry, fish, beans, and nuts, creates a harmonious balance that sustains energy levels and supports muscle function.

Incorporating energy-boosting foods into your nutrition plan becomes a strategic investment in your well-being. Foods rich in iron, such as leafy greens, lean red meats, and fortified cereals, promote healthy oxygen transport in the body, reducing the risk of fatigue. Omega-3 fatty acids in fatty fish like salmon and flaxseeds enhance cognitive function and mental clarity. Including a variety of colorful fruits and vegetables provides essential vitamins and minerals and infuses your diet with antioxidants that combat oxidative stress and enhance overall vitality.

Meal prep and snack planning are invaluable tools in ensuring sustained energy throughout the day. Preparing balanced meals in advance, rich in whole grains, lean proteins, and a rainbow of vegetables, eliminates the need to resort to quick, less-nutritious options during hectic hours. Consider whole-grain salads with grilled chicken, quinoa bowls loaded with vegetables and beans, or stir-fried tofu with vibrant stir-fried veggies. Snacks should be designed to stave off energy slumps between meals, combining protein, healthy fats, and fiber. Examples include Greek yogurt with berries and nuts, hummus and vegetable sticks, or whole-grain crackers with nut butter.

By understanding the pivotal role of nutrition in sustaining energy levels, you can empower yourself to tackle your daily tasks with vitality. Making thoughtful choices to include energy-boosting foods and engaging in strategic meal prep ensures that your body remains energized and ready to seize the day's challenges. Through this synergy of mindful nutrition and proactive planning, you set the stage for a life marked by vibrancy, productivity, and a profound sense of well-being.

Summary

In the fast-paced landscape of your life, the significance of energy mastery takes center stage. This chapter peels back the layers of energy, unraveling its impact on productivity, focus, and overall quality. From the vital role of various energy sources that encompass physical, mental, emotional, and spiritual realms to the strategic use of nutrition for fueling the body, the chapter illuminates the pathways to sustainable vitality.

Action Steps:

1. Energy Inventory: Take a closer look at your daily routines, identifying moments of peak and low energy levels. Document activities that contribute to rejuvenation and those that drain your energy. This self-awareness forms the basis for crafting an individualized energy-enhancing strategy.

2. Mindful Rejuvenation: Dedicate regular intervals to engage in mindful practices that recharge your mental energy, which could involve meditation, journaling, or pursuing a hobby that resonates with you. These moments of mental reprieve cultivate cognitive clarity and fortitude.

3. Nutritional Vitality: Review your dietary choices, ensuring the integration of energy-boosting foods. Enrich your meals with a blend of complex carbohydrates, lean proteins, and various fruits and vegetables. Aim for a combination of protein, healthy fats, and fiber for snacks to maintain consistent energy levels. What energy-rich foods are you going to add to your meal plan?

Navigating the diverse dimensions of energy without comparisons, this chapter unveils the power of strategic energy management. By comprehending the intricate interplay of physical, mental, and emotional vitality and harnessing the potential of nutrition, you chart a course toward a life marked by sustained energy, productivity, and a profound sense of well-being.

CHAPTER 4

Lunch Break Revitalization

Fueling Your Body for Maximum Workday Production

"In the pursuit of health and wellness, remember that small, consistent steps lead to remarkable transformations. Embrace the journey and celebrate every milestone along the way."
–Jody Dotson

In the fast-paced realm of modern workplaces, where time is often a precious commodity, nutrition emerges as an unsung hero that directly impacts the well-being and performance of busy working women. This chapter delves into the crucial role of nutrition within the workplace, exploring its significance in enhancing productivity, sustaining energy levels, and fostering overall health. From understanding the far-reaching effects of workplace nutrition to discovering practical snack ideas, this chapter aims to equip you with the knowledge and strategies to fuel your success from within.

The Importance of Workplace Nutrition

Nutrition is far more than a routine act of sustenance; it's a pivotal factor that underpins productivity, mental clarity, and physical vitality in the workplace. When you prioritize your nutritional intake, you equip yourself with the necessary tools to navigate the demands of your roles with efficacy and vigor. A balanced diet fuels cognitive function, allowing for sharper focus, better decision-making, and an enhanced ability to manage tasks efficiently. Moreover, when nourishing foods become a fundamental part of the workplace routine, energy levels remain steady throughout the day, preventing the dreaded mid-afternoon energy slumps that can hamper productivity.

However, the lack of attention to workplace nutrition can manifest in adverse ways. Skipping meals or opting for convenience foods high in sugar and refined carbohydrates may lead to energy crashes and diminished cognitive function. These dietary choices can contribute to feelings of irritability, reduced concentration, and decreased work performance. Furthermore, inadequate nutrition over time can impact overall health, increasing the risk of chronic diseases and compromising the body's resilience to stress. Neglecting nutrition in the workplace doesn't only affect individual well-being; it can have a ripple effect, impacting team dynamics, collaboration, and the overall work environment.

Snack Smart

Do you often find yourself navigating demanding schedules, leaving little room for elaborate meals? In such scenarios, strategically chosen snacks can become the pillars of energy and sustenance. Opt for snacks that provide a balance of nutrients, combining complex carbohydrates, protein, and healthy fats. Greek yogurt with berries and a sprinkle of nuts offers a blend of protein and antioxidants. A handful of mixed nuts and dried fruits deliver a combination of fiber and healthy fats. Fresh fruit paired with a small portion of cheese offers a delightful balance of flavors and nutrients. These snack options not only satiate hunger but also contribute to sustained energy levels, keeping you focused and productive throughout the workday.

As we venture to unravel the intricate dance between nutrition and the workplace, this chapter provides insights into the pivotal role of nourishment in enhancing performance and well-being. By embracing the wisdom of mindful nutritional choices and incorporating nourishing snacks, you empower yourself to thrive amidst the demands of your career. Through this harmonious integration of nutrition into the workplace routine, you carve a path toward a balanced and vibrant professional journey.

Summary

Within the bustling world of the workplace, nutrition emerges as a silent protagonist that influences your trajectory for success. This chapter unveils the multifaceted impact of workplace nutrition, shedding light on its role in elevating productivity, maintaining energy levels, and fostering overall well-being. By understanding the consequences of neglecting nutrition and embracing practical snack ideas, you are empowered to cultivate a thriving, nourishing environment within your professional life.

Action Steps:

1. Health and Wellness Assessment: Reflect on your current workplace nutrition habits. Are you regularly fueling your body with balanced meals and snacks, or do convenience foods dominate your choices? Take note of how your energy levels and performance are

affected by your dietary choices. Here is a link to a free assessment tool: https://forms.gle/KCmiHZTythBLQLKz7

2. Strategic Snacking: Plan ahead and prepare various nutrient-dense snacks you can quickly grab during your work-day. Include options that provide a mix of complex carbohydrates, protein, and healthy fats to sustain your energy levels and enhance focus. What smart snack options will you include?

3. Mindful Meal Breaks: Dedicate time for proper meal breaks. Use this time to consume balanced meals that incorporate a range of whole foods, supporting cognitive function and overall health. Steer clear of rushed or skipped meals that can lead to energy dips and decreased productivity. What is your lunchtime meal plan for this week?

By recognizing the pivotal role of nutrition within the workplace, you can create a foundation for sustained success and well-being. Embracing intentional nutritional choices and integrating nourishing snacks elevates personal performance and contributes to a positive and productive work environment. Through these transformative actions, you navigate your professional journey with resilience, focus, and a profound sense of vitality.

CHAPTER 5

Sugar Freedom

Empowering Yourself to Live a Healthier, Sweeter Life

"True health is a harmonious balance of the body, mind, and spirit, nourished by self-care and fueled by positive choices."
— Jody Dotson

In a world where sugar-laden temptations abound, the decision to detox from sugar emerges as a transformative step towards reclaiming your health. This chapter embarks on a journey of understanding the impact of sugar on your well-being and the remarkable benefits of a sugar detox. From unraveling the effects of sugar addiction to providing practical strategies for eliminating sugar from your kitchen and daily routine, this chapter is a comprehensive guide to embarking on a sugar-free lifestyle that nurtures vitality and well-being.

The Effects of Sugar

The allure of sugar is undeniable - its sweetness can be tantalizing, comforting, and momentarily gratifying. Yet, beneath its appealing exterior lies a bitter truth that impacts your body in profound ways. Sugar addiction, often underestimated, operates like a relentless cycle, contributing to a myriad of health concerns that stretch far beyond the waistline. It operates in cycles that leave a trail of consequences on your body and mind. The perils of excessive sugar consumption extend beyond the well-known risk of weight gain to encompass increased risks of chronic diseases such as diabetes, heart disease, and even mental health issues. Unraveling hidden sugars that lurk in seemingly innocent foods becomes essential to regaining control over your dietary choices. From the sneaky additives in packaged snacks to the sweet traps in condiments, recognizing these sources empowers you to make informed decisions.

Sugar triggers a cascade of biochemical reactions in the brain, releasing dopamine, a neurotransmitter associated with pleasure. This initial euphoria soon fades, leaving you craving that same pleasurable sensation. Consequently, the cycle of consuming sugar to chase that fleeting high begins, leading to a rollercoaster of cravings and overconsumption. This addiction cycle not only disrupts your relationship with food but can also result in weight gain, insulin resistance, and even mood swings.

The impact of excessive sugar consumption extends beyond the concern of weight gain. Regularly indulging in sugary treats can lead to insulin resistance, a precursor to diabetes, as your body struggles to manage blood sugar levels effectively. Furthermore, the inflammation caused by excess sugar in your bloodstream increases the risk of chronic diseases such as heart disease and certain types of cancer. Moreover, sugar can wreak havoc on your skin, accelerating the aging process and contributing to skin conditions like acne.

Unveiling the hidden sugars that hide in everyday foods is a vital step towards taking control of your health. Many seemingly healthy products, from yogurt to salad dressings, can contain astonishing amounts of added sugars. Learning to read nutrition labels becomes an essential skill, as various disguises for sugar may include terms like high fructose corn syrup, cane sugar, or even evaporated cane juice. By recognizing these hidden sources, you empower yourself to make informed choices and reduce your sugar intake.

Understanding the effects of sugar on your body is not about vilifying this sweet substance entirely, but about acknowledging its potential impact and making conscious decisions. By recognizing the addictive cycle, understanding the health risks, and identifying hidden sugars, you gain the knowledge to navigate your dietary choices mindfully. This awareness forms the foundation for the transformative journey ahead - a journey towards a life free from the shackles of sugar's grasp and a state of balanced well-being and vitality.

Your Sugar Detox Blueprint

Participating in a sugar detox journey requires more than just a decision; it necessitates a well-thought-out plan that empowers you to navigate the challenges and triumphs along the way. Creating a sugar detox blueprint involves setting clear intentions, enlisting support, preparing your environment, and equipping yourself with strategies to stay on track when faced with inevitable temptations.

Begin your sugar detox by defining your goals with clarity. Are you aiming to reduce sugar intake, eliminate refined sugars, or fully detox from all sources of added sugars? Your goals will serve as your guiding light, providing a sense of purpose and direction as you progress. Be specific about what you want to achieve: increased energy, weight loss, better skin, or improved overall well-being. These objectives will serve as reminders of your purpose, motivating you to stay committed even when the path gets challenging.

Enlist the support of friends, family, or online communities that share your health goals. Having a support system provides a network of accountability, encouragement, and shared experiences. Share your intentions with those close to you, allowing them to understand and respect your dietary choices. Additionally, joining online groups or seeking out a mentor who has successfully completed a sugar detox can offer insights, tips, and the reassurance that you're not on this journey alone.

Prepare for your sugar detox by equipping yourself with nourishing meal options. Meal prepping saves time and ensures you have wholesome, sugar-free choices readily available. Prioritize whole foods such as vegetables, lean proteins, whole grains, and healthy fats to fuel your body while minimizing cravings. While planning is essential, it's equally important to acknowledge that setbacks can happen. Having a backup plan for when you slip up ensures you can swiftly get back on track without entirely derailing your progress.

Approach your sugar detox journey with a positive mindset. View it as an opportunity to nurture your body and embark on a transformative path toward improved health. Embrace the potential challenges as opportunities for growth and learning. Celebrate your victories, no matter how small, and practice self-compassion if you encounter setbacks. By fostering a positive outlook, you create a fertile ground for sustainable change and a healthier relationship with food.

Your sugar detox blueprint serves as your roadmap to a healthier, sugar-free lifestyle. By setting clear goals, surrounding yourself with a supportive community, preparing your environment, and maintaining a positive mindset, you lay the foundation for lasting change. As you take these proactive steps, you empower yourself to embark on a transformative journey that celebrates the beauty of mindful choices and the vitality that comes with embracing a sugar-free life.

Say Goodbye to Sugar

The decision to embrace a sugar-free lifestyle marks a significant shift in how you nourish your body and engage with food. As you bid farewell to sugar, you embark on a journey of reimagining your kitchen, revamping your meals, and exploring the realm of sugar substitutes that offer the sweetness you crave without the detrimental effects of refined sugar.

Begin your sugar-free journey by conducting a thorough audit of your kitchen. Remove items that contain added sugars or high amounts of hidden sweeteners. Say goodbye to sugary cereals, flavored yogurts, bottled sauces, and processed snacks that often harbor excess sugars. Replace these items with nutrient-dense alternatives that align with your goals of reducing sugar intake. Whole foods like whole grains, lean proteins, fresh vegetables, and healthy fats become the building blocks of your sugar-free kitchen.

With sugar no longer occupying a prominent role in your diet, you have the opportunity to explore an array of flavors and ingredients. Embrace the natural sweetness of whole foods like fruits, vegetables, and grains. For example, have you ever tried nice cream? Blend strawberries or bananas with plant-based milk in a blender. When it is smooth, place the blended mixture into the freezer and let it chill. Nice cream is a healthy alternative to ice cream. Experiment with different herbs, spices, and seasoning blends to enhance the taste of your meals without relying on added sugars. As you create meals that nourish your body and palate, you'll likely discover a renewed appreciation for the rich tapestry of flavors that real, unprocessed foods offer.

While eliminating refined sugars, it's natural to seek alternatives that provide the sweetness you enjoy. Natural sugar substitutes such as stevia, different fruits, and erythritol (a sugar substitute) can be integrated into your recipes and beverages. These alternatives offer the satisfaction of sweetness without causing dramatic spikes in blood sugar levels. However, it's important to use them in moderation and be mindful of their impact on your body. Gradually reduce your dependence on sweeteners over time to recalibrate your taste buds and appreciate the innate sweetness of whole foods.

Designing a meal plan that aligns with your sugar-free goals is pivotal to your success. Incorporate various nutrient-dense foods to ensure you receive a balanced array of vitamins, minerals, and macronutrients. Prepare meals ahead of time to avoid reaching for sugary convenience options when hunger strikes. Whether you're whipping up colorful salads, protein-rich stir-fries, or hearty grain bowls, your meal plan becomes a roadmap that guides you toward nourishment, satisfaction, and wellness.

Saying goodbye to sugar opens the door to a fresh chapter of culinary exploration and holistic well-being. By purging your pantry, embracing whole foods, experimenting with natural sweeteners, and crafting a thoughtful meal plan, you sculpt an environment that fosters nourishment and vitality. As you embark on this journey, remember that every meal prepared in your revamped kitchen is an act of self-love, nurturing your body and honoring your commitment to a sugar-free lifestyle.

Surviving Withdrawal and Overcoming Challenges

As you start your sugar detox journey, it's important to anticipate and address the challenges that may arise. From the withdrawal symptoms that might test your resolve to the social situations that tempt your commitment, understanding these challenges and developing strategies to navigate them is essential for your success in embracing a sugar-free lifestyle.

Withdrawal from sugar can trigger a range of symptoms as your body adjusts to the absence of its accustomed sweet indulgence. These symptoms may include headaches, mood swings, fatigue, and intense cravings. Remember that these sensations are temporary and are indicative of your body recalibrating itself. Stay hydrated, prioritize nutrient-dense foods, and engage in stress-relief practices such as deep breathing, meditation, or light exercise to alleviate the discomfort. Recognizing that these symptoms are a sign of progress can empower you to persevere through this challenging phase.

Sugar cravings can be overwhelming, especially in the initial stages of your sugar detox. To address these cravings, adopt proactive strategies that help redirect your focus and manage the urges. Keep nutrient-dense snacks readily available to satiate hunger and prevent reaching for sugary treats. Engage in mindful activities such as taking a short walk, practicing deep breathing, or enjoying a warm herbal tea to curb cravings. Over time, as your body adjusts to a sugar-free lifestyle, you'll likely find that these cravings diminish, and your taste buds recalibrate to appreciate the natural sweetness of whole foods.

Navigating social situations and dining out can present challenges to your sugar detox efforts. When faced with a spread of sugary treats or invitations to indulge, take a proactive approach. Communicate your dietary preferences to friends and family, helping them understand your commitment to a sugar-free lifestyle. Consider offering to bring a dish or dessert that aligns with your goals. When dining out, choose restaurants with diverse menu options that allow you to make choices that suit your dietary preferences. Focus on enjoying the company and conversation rather than solely on the food, shifting your perspective from restriction to empowerment.

Approaching the challenges of withdrawal and social eating with a resilient mindset is fundamental to your success. Embrace the notion that challenges are opportunities for growth and self-discovery. Be patient with yourself, recognizing that progress is not linear and slip-ups are part of the journey. If you give in to a sweet treat, don't overindulge. Recommit to your goals and keep moving forward. Cultivate self-compassion and celebrate your achievements, no matter how small. By nurturing a resilient mindset, you equip yourself with the tools to overcome obstacles, stay committed to sugar-free goals, and emerge stronger and more empowered than ever before.

Summary

In this chapter, you've uncovered the multifaceted impact of sugar on your health and gained insights into embarking on a sugar detox journey. From understanding sugar addiction cycles to setting clear goals and strategies, you're equipped with the tools to embrace a sugar-free lifestyle. By reimagining your kitchen, navigating withdrawal symptoms, and confidently approaching social eating, you pave the way for lasting well-being and vitality.

Action Steps:

1. Take the Sugar Quiz: See where you are with sugar. Use the link to take a free sugar quiz: https://forms.gle/nxGw9e9QxxeKVR6E9.
2. Define Your Goals: Reflect on why you want to eliminate sugar from your diet. Set specific and achievable goals that will guide your journey.
3. Create a Support System: Share your intentions with friends or family who can offer encouragement. Join online groups for additional motivation.
4. Plan Your Meals: Devote time to meal prep and stock your kitchen with sugar-free options. What is going to be your sugar-free go-to when you are craving something sweet?

CHAPTER 6

Reversing Chronic Illness
The Lifestyle Medicine Approach

"By cleansing your body on a regular basis and eliminating as many toxins as possible from your environment, your body can begin to heal itself, prevent disease, and become stronger and more resilient than you ever dreamed possible!"
– Dr. Edward Group III

The intricate relationship between diet, nutrition, and chronic illness is a dynamic terrain that impacts our bodies and quality of life. This chapter delves into the profound connection between what we consume and the trajectory of chronic illnesses, shedding light on how nutrition can serve as a potent tool for both managing and potentially reversing the course of these conditions. From understanding the core role of nutrition in chronic illness progression to exploring personalized dietary approaches, this chapter serves as a comprehensive guide to harnessing the power of nutrition for a journey toward wellness.

The Role of Nutrition in Chronic Illness

To comprehend the significance of nutrition in the realm of chronic illness, it's imperative to grasp the multifaceted factors contributing to the onset and progression of these conditions. Chronic illnesses are often rooted in a combination of genetic predisposition, lifestyle factors, environmental exposures, and inflammation. Nutrition plays a pivotal role in influencing inflammation levels, oxidative stress, immune function, and gut health - all of which are intertwined with the development and course of chronic diseases.

Chronic illnesses arise from a myriad of factors, each contributing to the intricate puzzle that shapes their manifestation. Genetic predisposition can set the stage for certain conditions, while lifestyle choices such as diet, physical activity, stress management, and sleep patterns can trigger or mitigate their progression. Environmental exposures, ranging from pollutants to infectious agents, further compound the complexity. Chronic symptoms, often diverse and wide-ranging, reflect the nuanced ways in which these underlying factors interact and impact the body.

At the heart of this complex system lies nutrition, a factor that can either fan the flames of inflammation or quell their intensity. The foods we consume have a direct impact on oxidative stress, immune function, gut health, and overall inflammation levels - all of which are intricately tied to chronic illness development. Highly processed foods laden with sugars, unhealthy fats, and artificial additives can contribute to inflammation, exacerbate symptoms, and fuel the progression of chronic conditions. On the other hand, a diet rich in nutrient-dense whole foods can provide the body with the tools it needs to combat inflammation, repair cellular damage, and promote healing.

Navigating the realm of chronic illness and nutrition necessitates acknowledging the unique landscape of each individual's health. Personalized nutrition approaches recognize that no two bodies are alike, and dietary needs should be tailored to one's specific health profile. Factors such as genetic predisposition, existing health conditions, nutrient deficiencies, and food sensitivities, play a pivotal role in shaping the ideal dietary approach. Through personalized nutrition, you can optimize your dietary choices to align with your unique needs, enhancing the potential for healing and wellness.

In the complicated interplay between chronic illness and nutrition, it's evident that the foods we choose to consume are not passive actors but active agents shaping our health trajectory. By grasping the complex nature of chronic illnesses and understanding how nutrition interacts with their development and progression, we embark on a journey of empowerment. The choices we make at the dining table resonate far beyond the immediate moment, influencing the very course of our well-being. As we unravel the threads of this complex web, we stand at the intersection of opportunity and transformation, armed with the knowledge that our nutritional choices have the power to mend, rejuvenate, and elevate our health.

Assessing Your Foundations

Assessing your current diet and lifestyle is a foundational step towards reclaiming your health. Reflect on your eating habits, identifying areas where processed foods, excess sugar, and unhealthy fats might be contributing to inflammation and exacerbating chronic symptoms. Simultaneously, evaluate lifestyle factors such as physical activity, stress management, and sleep quality that can significantly influence the progression of chronic conditions. Maintaining a food journal can shed light on potential triggers for symptoms, providing valuable insights into patterns and connections between diet and health.

Start by casting a discerning eye on your eating habits. Reflect on the types of foods you regularly consume, the portion sizes, and the frequency of meals and snacks throughout the day. Are processed foods, sugary beverages, or high-sodium options dominant in your diet? Recognizing these dietary patterns and identifying areas where you might be consuming excess sugars, unhealthy fats, or artificial additives is essential in understanding how your diet might be contributing to inflammation and exacerbating chronic symptoms.

Beyond your diet, other lifestyle factors contribute to your overall health and the progression of chronic illnesses. Reflect on your physical activity levels, stress management techniques, sleep quality, and exposure to environmental toxins. Inadequate exercise, high stress levels, poor sleep patterns, and exposure to pollutants can all contribute to inflammation and hinder your efforts to manage chronic conditions. Acknowledging these factors provides a comprehensive view of how your lifestyle might be influencing your health.

One of the most powerful tools at your disposal is keeping a food journal. Document your daily meals, snacks, beverages, and any symptoms you experience. This practice helps you establish connections between your diet and the onset or exacerbation of chronic symptoms. Note any changes in energy levels, digestive issues, skin conditions, or mood fluctuations. Over time, patterns may emerge, shedding light on potential triggers and helping you make informed choices about the foods you consume.

Assessing your dietary foundations isn't about blame or judgment; it's about equipping yourself with the knowledge to make positive changes. As you evaluate your eating habits and lifestyle factors, you'll gain insight into the areas that require adjustment and transformation. By embracing your blueprint for change, you're setting the stage for a holistic approach to wellness that considers not only what you eat but how you nourish your body and support its healing journey.

Navigating Wellness Through Nutrition: Supporting Chronic Illness with Nutrient-Dense Foods

Certain nutrients emerge as champions in the journey toward chronic illness reversal. Antioxidants, omega-3 fatty acids, fiber, and a variety of vitamins and minerals are vital for reducing inflammation, supporting immune function, and promoting overall health. Fruits, vegetables, fatty fish, nuts, seeds, and whole grains become the building blocks of a nutrient-rich foundation. These foods collectively supply the body with the tools it needs to combat oxidative stress, repair cellular damage, and foster an environment conducive to healing.

Nutrition serves as the cornerstone of your healing journey. By adopting a nutrient-dense diet, you provide your body with the building blocks it needs to repair and regenerate. Whole, unprocessed foods brimming with vitamins, minerals, antioxidants, and phytonutrients offer the raw materials required for cellular rejuvenation. Incorporating a colorful array of fruits and vegetables, lean or plant-based proteins, whole grains, and healthy fats fosters an environment conducive to recovery and vitality.

Balancing macronutrients—carbohydrates, proteins, and fats—forms a fundamental aspect of your nutritional approach. Complex carbohydrates supply sustained energy, fiber for gut health, and essential nutrients. Adequate protein intake supports tissue repair and immune function. Meanwhile, healthy fats, such as those found in avocados, nuts, and fatty fish, aid in nutrient absorption and provide anti-inflammatory benefits. Crafting meals that harmoniously combine these macronutrients promotes stable blood sugar levels, reduces inflammation, and supports overall wellness.

Hydration, often overlooked, plays a pivotal role in your healing journey. Water serves as a medium for essential biochemical reactions and aids in detoxification. Adequate hydration promotes optimal digestion, circulation, and cellular function. Infuse your day with hydrating herbal teas, infused waters, and nourishing broths to support your body's healing mechanisms.

While a nutrient-dense diet forms the foundation, targeted supplementation can offer additional support. Deficiencies in certain vitamins and minerals, common in chronic illness, can hinder your progress. Collaborate with healthcare professionals to identify specific needs and incorporate supplements that enhance your body's capacity to heal.

Parallel to nutrition, lifestyle enhancements work synergistically to propel your healing journey. Adequate sleep restores cellular function, while physical activity improves circulation, mood, and overall well-being. Mindfulness practices, such as meditation and deep breathing, soothe stress and reduce inflammation. Engaging in meaningful social connections and nurturing a positive outlook can fortify your mental and emotional resilience.

By crafting a nutrient-rich foundation rooted in whole foods, balanced macronutrients, hydration, and targeted supplementation, you provide your body with the tools it needs to reverse chronic illness and thrive. Complemented by lifestyle enhancements, this holistic approach fosters a transformational environment where healing can flourish. Your journey toward optimal health is uniquely your own, and by embracing these key elements, you empower your body's innate ability to heal and reclaim vitality.

Designing a Healing Meal Plan

Creating a meal plan that incorporates nutrient-dense foods is pivotal in orchestrating your chronic illness reversal journey. Start your day with a balanced breakfast that includes protein, healthy fats, and fiber to stabilize blood sugar levels. Prioritize lean or plant-based proteins, colorful vegetables, whole grains, and healthy fats throughout the day to fuel your body with the necessary nutrients. Hydration is equally vital - consume water, herbal teas, and hydrating foods to support cellular function and overall vitality.

Balance is the bedrock of a healing meal plan. Each meal should encompass a harmonious blend of macronutrients - proteins, carbohydrates, and healthy fats. Begin your day with a balanced breakfast that includes a source of lean or plant-based protein, such as eggs, tofu scramble, or Greek yogurt, paired with complex carbohydrates like whole grains and vibrant vegetables. Incorporate healthy fats from sources like avocados, nut butters, nuts, seeds, and olive oil to nourish your body and provide a slow, sustained release of energy.

A healing meal plan thrives on nutrient-dense foods that pack a powerful nutritional punch. Fruits and vegetables, rich in vitamins, minerals, and antioxidants, should grace your plate in a variety of colors. Dark leafy greens, vibrant berries, cruciferous vegetables, and citrus fruits infuse your body with antioxidants that combat inflammation and promote cellular repair. Incorporate lean proteins such as poultry, fish, legumes, and plant-based proteins such as legumes, tempeh, and tofu to support muscle function and immune health.

Whole grains are an essential component of a healing meal plan, providing sustained energy release and promoting digestive health. Opt for options like quinoa, brown rice, whole wheat, oats, and barley. These grains are rich in fiber, which supports gut function, regulates blood sugar levels, and contributes to a sense of fullness. Fiber also nourishes the beneficial gut bacteria, fostering a healthy gut environment that is intricately linked to overall well-being.

Water is a cornerstone of any healing meal plan. Hydration supports cellular function, aids digestion, and promotes detoxification. Infuse your day with water, herbal teas, and water-rich foods like cucumbers, watermelon, and leafy greens. Staying hydrated ensures your body can effectively transport nutrients, flush out toxins, and maintain optimal bodily functions.

Incorporating mindfulness into your meal plan can amplify its healing potential. Mindful eating involves savoring each bite, eating slowly, and tuning into your body's hunger and fullness cues. This practice not only enhances your enjoyment of food but also allows you to make intentional choices that align with your health goals. Cultivating mindfulness while eating can prevent overeating, improve digestion, and foster a deeper connection with your body's nutritional needs.

Designing a healing meal plan is not a one-size-fits-all endeavor; it's a dynamic process that evolves alongside your health journey. Regularly assess how your body responds to different foods, listen to its signals, and adjust your meal plan accordingly. Be open to experimenting with new ingredients, flavors, and cooking techniques to keep your meals exciting and nourishing. Through this ongoing customization, you create a meal plan that resonates with your body's needs and supports your ongoing pursuit of wellness.

Avoid Harmful Foods

In the pursuit of chronic illness reversal, it's crucial to identify and eliminate harmful foods that contribute to inflammation, exacerbate symptoms, and hinder progress. Processed foods laden with artificial additives, excessive sugar, refined grains, and unhealthy fats can perpetuate chronic inflammation and undermine your efforts. By learning how to identify these harmful foods and adopting strategies to avoid them, you cultivate a supportive environment for your body's healing journey.

Harmful foods are often characterized by their high content of added sugars, unhealthy fats, refined grains, artificial additives, and excess sodium. Processed foods, such as sugary cereals, packaged snacks, fast food, and sugary beverages, are prime examples of these detrimental culprits. These foods can lead to spikes in blood sugar levels, inflammation, oxidative stress, and disruptions in gut health - all of which can exacerbate chronic symptoms and hinder your journey toward wellness.

One of the most effective tools in your arsenal is the ability to decipher food labels. Prioritize whole foods that come with minimal or no packaging, and when you do opt for packaged items, diligently read labels. Look out for hidden sources of sugars (such as high fructose corn syrup and various syrups), unhealthy trans fats, and artificial additives. Ingredients listed towards the beginning of the label are present in larger quantities, so being aware of what you're consuming can guide you in making informed choices. Here are some key culprits to watch out for:

Added Sugars: Excessive sugar consumption has been linked to numerous health issues, including obesity and diabetes. Look for terms like high-fructose corn syrup, sucrose, and various syrups in the ingredient list. The American Heart Association recommends limiting added sugars to no more than 25 grams (about six teaspoons) per day for women and 36 grams (about nine teaspoons) for men.

Trans Fats: These are often found in partially hydrogenated oils and are a major contributor to heart disease. The goal is to avoid them entirely. Check the ingredient list for any mention of "partially hydrogenated" oils.

Sodium: Excess sodium can lead to high blood pressure and other health problems. Be mindful of the sodium content in processed foods, especially if you have a history of hypertension. In accordance with the *Dietary Guidelines for Americans*, it's advised to keep sodium intake below 2300 mg daily, which is equivalent to one teaspoon of salt.

Artificial Additives: Artificial flavors, colors, and preservatives can have adverse effects on health, particularly in individuals sensitive to these compounds. Opt for foods with minimal artificial additives or, better yet, none at all.

Highly Processed Ingredients: Foods with a long list of ingredients, especially those with names you can't pronounce, are often highly processed. These can be less nutritious and may contain hidden unhealthy components.

Unhealthy Fats: While not all fats are bad, it's essential to avoid or limit saturated and trans fats. Opt for foods that contain healthier fats, like monounsaturated and polyunsaturated fats.

Hidden Allergens: If you have food allergies or intolerances, thoroughly examine labels for any ingredients that may trigger an adverse reaction.

Calories and Serving Sizes: Pay attention to portion sizes and the number of calories per serving. It's easy to underestimate how many calories you consume if you're unaware of the serving size.

Reading food labels diligently helps equip you with the knowledge to make informed choices, ensuring you avoid these potential dietary pitfalls. Eating healthy is not only about what you include in your day-to-day meals but also what you exclude, making label scrutiny an essential tool in your quest for optimal well-being.

Processed foods often reside in the center aisles of grocery stores, while fresh produce, lean or plant-based proteins, and whole grains typically populate the periphery. By structuring your shopping around the periphery of the store, you naturally gravitate towards nutrient-dense options and minimize exposure to harmful additives. Fill your cart with colorful fruits, vegetables, whole grains, lean or plant-based proteins, and healthy fats to create a foundation that supports your healing journey.

Preparing meals at home offers a dual advantage - you have full control over the ingredients you use and gain a deeper connection to the foods that nourish you. Cooking at home allows you to select high-quality, whole ingredients while avoiding the hidden sugars, unhealthy fats, and additives often found in restaurants and fast-food options. Experimenting with different cooking techniques, herbs, and spices can enhance flavors without the need for excessive sugars or unhealthy additives.

Holistic Lifestyle Factors for Wellness

While nutrition is a cornerstone of chronic illness reversal, other lifestyle factors play an equally pivotal role. Prioritize regular physical activity, practice stress management techniques such as mindfulness and meditation, and ensure you're getting adequate sleep. These lifestyle elements synergize with nutrition to create a comprehensive wellness approach that promotes healing from within.

Regular physical activity isn't just a means to burn calories; it's a potent form of medicine that can alleviate symptoms, promote circulation, reduce inflammation, and enhance overall mood. Engage in activities that resonate with you, whether brisk walks, yoga, swimming, or dancing. Aim for a balanced routine that combines cardiovascular exercise, strength training, and flexibility exercises. Physical activity not only supports your body's healing journey but also fosters a sense of empowerment and vitality. It is understandable that committing to 150 minutes of weekly physical activity may seem like a substantial goal, but it doesn't have to be done in a single session. You have the flexibility to allocate 30 minutes a day, spread across five days a week. This way, you can distribute your exercise throughout the week and divide it into shorter, manageable segments of time. If time management is an issue, you can break down your 30 minutes into 15-minute exercises.

Stress, often a common companion of chronic illness, can significantly impact your health and well-being. Embracing stress management techniques, such as mindfulness meditation, deep breathing exercises, progressive muscle relaxation, and engaging in hobbies, can mitigate the effects of stress on your body. These practices foster a sense of calm, balance the nervous system, and positively influence hormone levels, ultimately contributing to better chronic illness management and overall wellness.

Sleep is a fundamental pillar of health, with profound implications for chronic illness management. Prioritize a consistent sleep schedule, creating a calming bedtime routine that signals to your body that it's time to unwind. Dim the lights, engage in relaxation practices, and avoid electronic screens before bed. Aim for seven to nine hours of quality sleep each night, as restorative sleep supports immune function, cellular repair, and mental clarity.

Your physical surroundings have a remarkable impact on your well-being. Declutter your space to reduce stress and promote mental clarity. Incorporate calming elements, such as indoor plants, soothing colors, and natural light, to create an environment that fosters relaxation and positivity. Cultivate mindfulness through practices like journaling, visualization, and grounding exercises, which connect your mind and body, enhancing your ability to manage chronic symptoms and navigate challenges.

Social connections play a pivotal role in your wellness journey. Engage with supportive friends, family members, and communities that understand

and respect your goals. Share your challenges and successes, seek advice, and offer your own insights. Participating in support groups, whether in-person or online, creates a sense of camaraderie, alleviates feelings of isolation, and provides a space to exchange experiences and coping strategies.

A balanced routine that encompasses physical activity, stress management, restful sleep, and nurturing environments amplifies the impact of your dietary efforts. By addressing your well-being from a holistic perspective, you're crafting an environment that promotes resilience, vitality, and a profound sense of empowerment in your health and wellness journey.

Collaborating with Healthcare Professionals

In your quest for chronic illness reversal, enlisting the guidance of health and wellness professionals is an invaluable step. Collaborating with a qualified nutritionist or dietitian, as well as effective communication with your health and wellness team (doctor, health coach, etc.), can provide personalized insights, tailored dietary recommendations, and ongoing support. Moreover, forging connections with support groups and online communities fosters a sense of camaraderie and shared experiences, enriching your wellness journey.

Navigating the complex terrain of chronic illness requires a multifaceted approach that extends beyond self-directed efforts. Healthcare professionals, including doctors, nutritionists, dietitians, and holistic health practitioners, bring a depth of knowledge to the table. They possess a nuanced understanding of how chronic conditions manifest, progress, and interact with dietary and lifestyle choices. By tapping into their expertise, you gain access to personalized insights that can guide your decisions, optimize your nutritional choices, and enhance your overall well-being.

Nutritionists and registered dietitians are adept at translating dietary recommendations into practical, actionable steps. Through comprehensive assessments, they can identify dietary patterns that contribute to chronic symptoms and develop customized meal plans that align with your health goals. These professionals factor in nutrient requirements, food sensitivities, allergies, and potential interactions with medications to create a plan that is not only effective but also sustainable for the long term. Collaborating with a nutrition expert empowers you to make informed choices and embark on a dietary journey that fosters optimal health.

A certified health and wellness coach, with a formal education, can play an essential role in guiding individuals toward better overall health and well-being. Their core responsibilities encompass:

- **Goal Establishment**: Collaborating with clients to identify their health and wellness objectives, encompassing weight management, stress reduction, nutrition enhancement, and fitness improvement.
- **Personalized Strategy**: Crafting tailored wellness plans that align with the client's specific requirements, preferences, and constraints. These plans often entail making lifestyle adjustments, modifying behaviors, and cultivating new habits.
- **Motivation and Accountability**: Offering continuous encouragement and support to help clients stay committed to their wellness aspirations, holding them responsible for their actions and advancements.
- **Informative Guidance**: Providing valuable insights and knowledge on diverse health facets, including nutrition, exercise, stress management, and sleep. Coaches empower clients to make informed decisions regarding their well-being.
- **Behavioral Transformation**: Assisting clients in identifying and surmounting obsta-

cles and unhealthy habits that impede their progress. Transformation of this kind involves nurturing healthier behaviors and effective coping strategies.

- **Progress Tracking**: Regularly monitoring and assessing clients' advancements toward their goals, making necessary adjustments to the wellness plan as required.
- **Emotional Support**: Extending emotional support and motivation, enabling clients to manage stress, anxiety, and other emotional factors that influence health.
- **Holistic Perspective**: Frequently adopting a holistic approach, recognizing the interconnectedness of physical, emotional, and mental well-being.
- **Referral and Collaboration**: In some instances, coaches may refer clients to other healthcare professionals when specialized care is essential, promoting a cooperative approach to holistic health.

A board-certified health and wellness coach, particularly geared towards women, serves as a steadfast partner in facilitating sustainable lifestyle transformations and the attainment of health and wellness objectives. They instill empowerment, enabling individuals to seize control of their health and lead lives that are healthier and more gratifying.

Effective collaboration with healthcare professionals involves open communication and a willingness to actively participate in your health journey. Share your health history, current symptoms, dietary habits, and lifestyle choices to provide a comprehensive picture of your well-being. Be receptive to their recommendations, ask questions, and clarify any doubts you may have. The synergy between your commitment and their guidance creates a dynamic partnership that propels you toward achieving your wellness goals.

In addition to individual consultations, consider participating in support groups and online communities that cater to individuals managing chronic illnesses. These groups provide a platform for sharing experiences, exchanging coping strategies, and seeking advice from those who understand your challenges firsthand. Engaging with these communities offers a sense of belonging, reduces feelings of isolation, and provides a space to ask questions and gather insights from a range of diverse perspectives.

Collaborating with healthcare professionals doesn't diminish your autonomy; rather, it empowers you to make informed decisions based on expert guidance. The insights you gain from these collaborations are tools that equip you with the knowledge and resources to steer your wellness journey with confidence. By valuing the expertise of healthcare professionals and engaging in proactive communication, you amplify your potential for positive outcomes, transformation, and a profound sense of well-being.

Summary

This chapter has illuminated the profound connection between nutrition and chronic illness, underscoring the potential for nutrition to shape the course of these conditions. From understanding the intricate factors that contribute to chronic illness to assessing your current diet and lifestyle, you're empowered with insights to steer your wellness journey. By embracing nutrient-rich foods, eliminating harmful culprits, and collaborating with healthcare professionals, you embark on a transformative path toward chronic illness reversal and holistic well-being.

Action Steps:

1. Self-Assessment: Reflect on your current diet and lifestyle. Identify areas for improvement, including sources of inflammation and potential triggers for chronic symptoms.

2. Food Journal Tracking: Keep a food journal to record your meals, snacks, and any symptoms experienced. This tracking can offer insights into patterns and connections between diet and health.

3. Hydration and Balanced Meals: Prioritize hydration and design balanced meals. How much water will you commit to drinking every day?

CHAPTER 7

Prioritizing You
Making Self-Care Non-negotiable

"Health is the foundation upon which we build our dreams, aspirations, and happiness. It is our most valuable asset; let us cherish and nurture it."
–Jody Dotson

With all of the distractions and demands in life today, it's easy to prioritize everything except yourself. Yet, amidst the demands of careers, relationships, and responsibilities, the practice of self-care emerges as an essential cornerstone of holistic well-being. This chapter delves into the heart of self-care, illuminating its multifaceted dimensions and providing a comprehensive guide to cultivating self-care practices that nourish the body, mind, and spirit.

Self-Care is a Multi-Dimensional Approach

Self-care is more than just an indulgence; it's a deliberate act of tending to your own needs to promote physical health, emotional well-being, and overall vitality. To do so requires encompassing various dimensions, each playing a unique role in your holistic wellness. Physical self-care rejuvenates your body through restful sleep, balanced nutrition, hydration, and regular exercise. Mental and emotional self-care involves managing stress, practicing mindfulness, and setting boundaries to safeguard your mental and emotional well-being. Spiritual self-care, often tied to meaning and purpose, involves engaging in practices that resonate with your inner self.

In a world that glorifies busyness, it's easy to fall into the trap of believing that self-care is a luxury, an indulgence reserved for those with an abundance of time and resources. However, this mindset fails to recognize the profound impact self-care can have on your overall well-being and, by extension, your ability to navigate the complexities of a busy life. Let's debunk these common misconceptions and unveil the truth about the accessibility and significance of self-care for busy working women.

The assertion that you don't have time for self-care is a paradoxical misconception. In reality, self-care isn't a drain on your time; it's an investment that yields returns in the form of increased focus, enhanced energy, and improved emotional resilience. Carving out moments for self-care doesn't demand a complete overhaul of your schedule. It can be as simple as a five-minute breathing exercise during a break or a brief mindfulness practice before starting your day. Recognizing that self-care need not be time-consuming reframes it as a series of intentional moments woven into your routine, enhancing your overall efficiency and well-being.

Another prevailing myth is that self-care requires substantial financial investment, an assumption that often discourages individuals from prioritizing their well-being. However, self-care isn't synonymous with lavish spa days or expensive retreats. It's about nurturing yourself in ways that resonate with you. Taking a leisurely walk, indulging in a book, practicing deep breathing exercises, or savoring a home-cooked meal can all be forms of self-care that cost nothing or very little. This shift in perspective liberates self-care from the confines of monetary resources; it empowers you to recognize that valuable self-care experiences are often found in the simplicity of daily life.

Perhaps the most pervasive misconception is the belief that self-care is an act of selfishness. This belief stems from a misconception that prioritizing your well-being takes away from others or that you don't deserve the time and attention you give to yourself. In truth, self-care is a fundamental necessity, not a luxury. Just as an empty vessel cannot pour into others, neglecting your well-being impedes your ability to be present, effective, and supportive in other aspects of your life. Cultivating self-care isn't an indulgence; it's an act of self-preservation and self-respect. Recognizing your worthiness to care for yourself is a pivotal shift that empowers you to become a stronger, more balanced version of yourself for both your own sake and for those you care about.

Challenging these misconceptions requires a shift in mindset that honors your well-being as an integral part of a fulfilling life. Embracing the accessibility of self-care, regardless of time or financial constraints, and acknowledging the inherent worthiness of nurturing yourself, transforms self-care from a fleeting concept to an empowering practice. By understanding that self-care is an investment in your physical, mental, and emotional well-being, you transcend the limitations of time and resources, allowing self-care to bloom as an enduring aspect of your daily life.

Nurturing Your Physical Well-being

Prioritizing physical self-care lays the foundation for holistic wellness. Adequate sleep, proper nutrition, and hydration are non-negotiable components. Aim for seven to nine hours of quality sleep, nourish your body with nutrient-dense foods, and stay hydrated. Incorporate regular physical activity that you enjoy, whether it's a morning walk, a dance class, or a yoga session, to invigorate your body and uplift your spirits.

With your busy schedule, sleep might seem like a negotiable commodity. However, sleep is a non-negotiable necessity that fuels your physical and mental faculties. Aim for seven to nine hours of uninterrupted sleep each night to allow your body to rejuvenate, repair, and restore. Create a tranquil sleep environment by minimizing electronic device usage before bed, dimming lights, and engaging in calming pre-sleep rituals. Prioritizing sleep not only enhances cognitive function and mood but also bolsters your immune system, helping you tackle challenges with resilience.

The foods you consume are the building blocks of your vitality. Embrace a balanced, nutrient-rich diet that fuels your body's needs. Prioritize whole foods such as fruits, vegetables, lean or plant-based proteins, whole grains, and healthy fats. Hydration is equally paramount; ensure you're drinking adequate water throughout the day to support digestion, circulation, and overall well-being. By viewing food as nourishment rather than mere convenience, you empower your body to thrive.

Adding regular physical activity into your routine can reap numerous benefits. Engage in exercises that resonate with you, whether it's jogging, dancing, yoga, or strength training. Exercise not only promotes cardiovascular health and strength but also boosts your mood by releasing endorphins. Aim for at least 150 minutes of moderate-intensity aerobic activity or 75 minutes of vigorous-intensity aerobic activity each week, complemented by muscle-strengthening activities on two or more days.

Begin by setting achievable goals. Allocate time for a daily brisk walk, engage in quick stretching breaks during your workday, or explore online workout classes that suit your schedule. Practice mindful eating by savoring each bite, choosing foods that nourish you, and avoiding emotional eating triggers. Keep a water bottle at hand as a reminder to stay hydrated throughout the day. By weaving these practices into your routine, you create a strong foundation that supports your physical vitality.

Prioritizing your physical well-being is not only an investment in your health but also a means of honoring your body's inherent resilience. As you embrace quality sleep, nourishing nutrition, and regular physical activity, you'll notice increased energy levels, improved focus, and a greater capacity to manage stress. Physical self-care equips you to thrive amidst challenges, empowering you to approach each day with strength and a sense of purpose.

Caring for Your Mental and Emotional Health

Managing stress becomes an art in itself. Engage in stress-reduction techniques such as mindfulness, meditation, and deep breathing exercises. Practice setting boundaries to protect your mental and emotional space and embrace the power of expressing your emotions in a healthy way. By acknowledging your feelings and seeking support when needed, you nurture your emotional well-being.

Stress is a constant companion in a busy working woman's life, but how you manage it makes all the difference. Begin by acknowledging your stress triggers and responses. Incorporate stress-reduction techniques such as deep breathing exercises, progressive muscle relaxation, and visualization to calm your nervous system and restore equilibrium. Regularly engage in activities that bring joy, whether it's reading, spending time in nature, or pursuing creative outlets. By proactively managing stress, you enhance your ability to navigate challenges and maintain emotional well-being.

Mindfulness and meditation offer powerful tools to cultivate awareness and presence. Carve out moments for mindfulness, even during a busy day. Engage in deep, conscious breathing exercises that ground you in the present moment. Incorporate meditation practices that resonate with you, whether it's guided meditation, body scans, or silent reflection. By anchoring yourself in the present, you release worries about the past or future, fostering a sense of calm and clarity.

Boundaries are your allies in maintaining mental and emotional equilibrium. Identify areas where you need to set boundaries to protect your time, energy, and emotional well-being. Learn to gracefully say no when necessary and prioritize activities that align with your values and goals. Embrace emotional intelligence by allowing yourself to experience and express your feelings in a healthy way. Whether it's through journaling, talking to a trusted friend, or engaging in creative outlets, expressing emotions frees you from their grip and nurtures emotional resilience.

Caring for your mental and emotional health isn't a luxury; it's an investment that yields a wealth of rewards. As you manage stress, practice mindfulness, set boundaries, and embrace emotional authenticity, you forge a path toward emotional resilience and well-being. These practices empower you to handle challenges with poise, cultivate meaningful connections, and approach life's ups and downs with a sense of balance and grace.

Creating a Supportive Environment

Crafting a supportive environment enhances your self-care journey. Declutter your physical space to create a sense of calm and clarity. Surround yourself with positive people and cultivate healthy relationships that uplift and empower you. Setting boundaries with your time and energy safeguards your well-being, allowing you to give to others while preserving your energy.

Physical clutter can weigh down not only your surroundings but also your mental and emotional state. Begin by decluttering your physical space, creating an environment that promotes clarity and tranquility. Set aside time to organize your belongings, letting go of items that no longer serve a purpose. A clutter-free environment reduces stress, enhances focus, and creates a canvas for intentional living. As you clear your physical space, you pave the way for mental clarity and emotional ease.

Your social circle significantly influences your well-being. Cultivate relationships with individuals who uplift, inspire, and support you on your journey. Surround yourself with people who encourage your growth, validate your feelings, and celebrate your successes. Nurture connections that align with your values and empower you to become the best version of yourself. The energy of positive connections amplifies your overall well-being, offering a network of support and understanding.

Establishing boundaries is a powerful form of self-care that protects your time, energy, and emotional well-being. Learn to say no when needed, prioritize your needs, and communicate your boundaries assertively but respectfully. By setting boundaries, you create a framework that shields you from overwhelm and burnout. Whether it's in your professional or personal life, clear boundaries empower you to focus on what truly matters and nurture your well-being.

Setting boundaries extends to maintaining a healthy work-life balance. Clearly define work hours and off-hours and resist the urge to constantly check emails or messages. Engage in activities that bring joy and fulfillment outside of work, whether it's spending time with loved ones, pursuing hobbies, or simply enjoying moments of solitude. By protecting your time and energy, you cultivate an environment that supports your overall well-being.

Crafting a supportive environment isn't merely about aesthetics; it's about creating a sanctuary that nurtures your growth, fosters your relationships, and shields you from unnecessary stress. As you declutter, curate connections, and set boundaries, you cultivate an environment that empowers your self-care journey. This environment becomes a refuge where you can recharge, align with your values, and manifest a life of authenticity and well-being.

Embracing Self-Love

Practicing self-love is at the heart of self-care. Accept yourself, imperfections and all, and extend kindness to yourself during challenging times. Celebrate your achievements, no matter how small, and practice gratitude for the present moment. This self-compassion enriches your well-being, fostering a sense of wholeness and empowerment.

Embracing self-love begins with self-acceptance—the practice of acknowledging and honoring your authentic self one hundred percent. Release the expectation of perfection and replace it with an embrace of your uniqueness. Treat yourself with the same kindness and compassion you extend to others. By embracing self-acceptance, you cultivate a resilient foundation that shields you from self-criticism and nurtures a sense of inner peace.

Self-love becomes particularly crucial during challenging times. Instead of neglecting your well-being when facing difficulties, practice self-care as a form of self-compassion. Engage in activities that soothe your spirit, whether it's journaling, taking walks, or seeking support from loved ones. By caring for yourself during trying moments, you foster resilience and empower yourself to weather life's storms with grace.

As you navigate the journey of self-love, remember to celebrate your achievements, both big and small. Often, busy women tend to downplay their successes, brushing them aside in pursuit of the next goal. However, taking time to acknowledge your achievements and milestones cultivates a sense of accomplishment and confidence. Celebrate each step forward, relishing the progress you've made on your self-care journey. Practice gratitude for your growth and the opportunity to nurture your well-being.

Practicing gratitude is a cornerstone of self-love. Acknowledge the blessings in your life, whether they're material, emotional, or relational. Dedicate moments each day to reflect on what you're grateful for and savor the positive experiences that enrich your life. By focusing on the abundance in your life, you shift your perspective and infuse your days with positivity and contentment.

Embracing self-love isn't a self-indulgent act; it's a transformative gift that empowers you to become the architect of your own well-being. By practicing self-acceptance, nurturing self-care during challenges, and celebrating your achievements with gratitude, you cultivate a sense of wholeness and worthiness. This self-love radiates outward, positively impacting your relationships, work, and every facet of your life.

Cultivating Social Connection and Community Care

Nurturing your connections with others is an integral aspect of self-care. Engage in meaningful conversations, spend quality time with loved ones, and engage in acts of kindness that contribute to your own and others' well-being. Building or connecting to a support network offers a safety net of encouragement and understanding during triumphs and trials.

Investing time and energy in meaningful relationships is a cornerstone of self-care. Prioritize spending quality moments with loved ones, engaging in heartfelt conversations, and fostering connections that uplift and empower you. Whether it's friends, family, or colleagues, these connections offer emotional support, understanding, and a sense of belonging that can lighten your load and infuse your life with joy.

Engaging in acts of kindness, whether big or small, is a powerful way to nurture your own well-being and contribute positively to the world around you. Acts of kindness need not be grand gestures; even a thoughtful message, a helping hand, or a simple compliment can create ripples of positivity. By giving back, you experience a profound sense of fulfillment and purpose and inspire others to do the same. These acts of kindness collectively weave a tapestry of compassion that strengthens your connection to your community.

Building or connecting to a support network enhances your resilience in the face of life's challenges. Engage with groups, organizations, or online communities that align with your interests and values. These networks provide a platform for sharing experiences, exchanging advice, and finding solace in the understanding of others who share similar experiences. Whether navigating work-related stress, personal struggles, or simply seeking camaraderie, support networks offer a source of comfort and encouragement.

Community care extends beyond your immediate circle to encompass the broader community you're a part of. Engaging in acts that contribute positively to your community, whether it's volunteering, participating in local initiatives, or supporting causes close to your heart, creates a reciprocal relationship of care and enrichment. As you give, you receive a sense of purpose and connection that reverberates, creating a more compassionate and thriving environment for all.

Cultivating social connection and community care isn't just a matter of self-care; it's a means of crafting a legacy of empathy, kindness, and positive change. By nurturing relationships, engaging in acts of kindness, and contributing to your community, you leave a lasting impact on the lives of those around you. This interconnectedness weaves a tapestry of resilience, nurturing the well-being of both yourself and the world you inhabit.

Summary

The art of self-care for busy working women is a journey of intention, balance, and empowerment. Embracing physical, mental, emotional, and spiritual dimensions creates a comprehensive approach to well-being. By dismantling misconceptions, embracing self-love, cultivating a supportive environment, and nurturing social connections, you create a harmonious symphony of self-care that resonates through every aspect of your life.

Action Steps:

1. Prioritize Sleep: Set a sleep routine to ensure seven to nine hours of quality sleep each night for revitalized energy.
2. Mindful Moments: Dedicate a few minutes each day to mindfulness or meditation to reduce stress and enhance clarity.
3. Create Boundaries: Identify areas where you need to set boundaries to protect your well-being and implement them with confidence.

CONCLUSION

As we come to the close of this transformative journey, it's clear that the threads of well-being extend far beyond individual chapters. Your journey through these pages has been a testament to the power of embracing a comprehensive approach to wellness—one that nurtures not only your physical health but also your mental clarity, emotional resilience, and self-compassion.

From debunking the myths of traditional diets to understanding the profound impact of stress, from naturally restoring your energy to removing sugar from your daily diet, you've explored a diverse range of topics that form the foundation of a well-balanced life. The wisdom gained from managing stress, revitalizing your energy, and cultivating healthy nutritional habits has equipped you with the tools to navigate the complexities of a busy life with grace and intention.

The chapters dedicated to reversing chronic illness through nutrition and lifestyle practices serve as a beacon of hope, illustrating the potential for transformation even in the face of adversity. Your journey toward holistic wellness is a testament to the resilience of the human spirit and the remarkable capacity of the body to heal when provided with the right nourishment and care.

The importance of self-care has been a recurring theme, reminding you that you are deserving of the same kindness and compassion that you extend to others. By cultivating self-love, setting boundaries, and nurturing positive connections, you've embraced the essence of well-being as a journey of self-discovery and empowerment.

As you close this chapter, remember that your wellness is an ongoing work of art—a canvas that evolves with each intentional choice you make. You possess the knowledge and tools to craft a life that resonates with strength, balance, and fulfillment. The journey toward holistic and nutritional wellness is not a destination but a continuous voyage, a dance of self-discovery, growth, and self-care that unfolds with each passing day.

As you move forward, let your journey be a living example of empowered wellness. Every step you take and every choice you make contributes to your well-being story. The essence of holistic and nutritional wellness is a gift you give yourself—one that brightens all areas of your life with health, balance, and a sense of fulfillment. Your path is a testament to your empowered, intentional, and wholehearted approach to living life to the fullest.

BONUS #1: HEALTHY SNACK SUGGESTIONS

1. Fresh Fruit: Sliced apples, pears, berries (raspberries, blueberries, and strawberries), or a banana are great choices.

2. Greek Yogurt: Opt for plain, unsweetened Greek yogurt and add a drizzle of honey or fresh fruit for flavor.

3. Raw Nuts: Almonds, walnuts, and cashews are excellent sources of healthy fats and protein.

4. Hummus and Veggies: Sliced cucumbers, bell peppers, carrot sticks, or celery with a side of hummus make for a satisfying and nutritious snack.

5. Whole Grain Crackers: Look for crackers with minimal ingredients and pair them with natural nut butter or cheese.

6. Hard-Boiled Eggs: Hard-boiled eggs are a protein-packed, portable snack.

7. Popcorn: Air-popped or made by stovetop popcorn is a whole grain option.

8. Cherry Tomatoes with Mozzarella: Combine cherry tomatoes with small mozzarella balls, drizzle with balsamic vinegar, and sprinkle with basil for a flavorful, low-calorie snack.

9. Oatmeal: A small bowl of oats with a touch of honey and some fresh fruit can be a wholesome snack.

10. Cottage Cheese: Cottage cheese is rich in protein and pairs well with fruit or a sprinkle of black pepper.

11. Avocado Toast: Spread mashed avocado on whole-grain toast and top with a pinch of sea salt or a drizzle of olive oil.

12. Rice Cakes: Top rice cakes with almond butter, sliced banana, or even a sprinkle of chia seeds.

13. Homemade Smoothies: Blend up a smoothie using fresh or frozen fruits, Greek yogurt, and a handful of spinach for added nutrients.

14. Sliced Cucumber with Tzatziki: Dip cucumber slices in homemade or low-sodium store-bought tzatziki sauce.

15. Roasted Chickpeas: Season chickpeas with your choice of spices and roast them for a crunchy, protein-packed snack.

16. Sliced Bell Peppers with Guacamole: Enjoy the crunch of bell peppers with a side of guacamole for healthy fats.

17. Dark Chocolate: In moderation, dark chocolate (70% cocoa or higher) can satisfy your sweet tooth.

18. Seeds: Pumpkin, chia, or sunflower seeds are nutrient-dense and can be eaten as a snack or added to yogurt or oatmeal.

19. Sliced Jicama: This crunchy, slightly sweet root vegetable is refreshing and low in calories.

20. Kale Chips: Homemade kale chips are a nutritious alternative to traditional potato chips.

21. These snacks offer a balance of macronutrients, vitamins, and minerals, while also being free from processed and

unhealthy additives, making them ideal choices for those striving to eat clean and stay healthy.

BONUS #2: SUGAR-FREE MEALS

Breakfast: Sugar-free oatmeal with Fresh Berries
Serves 2

Ingredients:

- 1/2 cup old-fashioned rolled oats
- 1 cup unsweetened almond milk (or your preferred milk)
- 1/2 teaspoon ground cinnamon
- 1/2 teaspoon pure vanilla extract
- Fresh mixed berries (strawberries, blueberries, raspberries, or any of your choice)
- Chopped nuts (almonds, walnuts, or pecans)
- Unsweetened shredded coconut (optional)
- Honey or a sugar-free sweetener like stevia (optional for added sweetness)

Instructions:

1. In a small saucepan, combine the rolled oats and almond milk. Heat the mixture over medium heat.

2. Stir in the ground cinnamon and pure vanilla extract. These ingredients will add flavor without in place of sugar.

3. Cook the oatmeal according to the instructions on the oatmeal package you selected, usually for about five to seven minutes, stirring occasionally. Adjust the amount of milk to achieve your desired consistency (to make it thicker, add more milk).

4. Once the oatmeal is cooked to your liking and has thickened, remove it from the heat and let it sit for a minute to cool slightly.

5. While the oatmeal is cooling, prepare your fresh mixed berries. Wash and slice them to your preference.

6. Scoop the desired amount of sugar-free oatmeal into a bowl

7. Top the oatmeal with the fresh mixed berries and chopped nuts.

8. If you desire extra sweetness, drizzle a small amount of honey.

Now, it is time to enjoy. This breakfast is not only sugar-free but is also packed with fiber, vitamins, and antioxidants from the fresh berries, making it a tasty and healthy way to start your day. Feel free to customize it with your favorite fruits and nuts to suit your preferences.

Lunch: Greek Salad with Lentils or Salmon
Serves 2

Ingredients:

- ¼ cup extra virgin olive oil
- 3 tablespoons raw apple cider vinegar or balsamic vinegar
- 1 teaspoon dried oregano
- sea salt and black pepper, to taste
- 2 cups spring mix
- 1 small cucumber, chopped
- ½ red onion, chopped
- ¼ cup olives, pitted
- 2 ripe tomatoes, sliced
- ¼ cup roasted red bell peppers from a jar and drained
- 4 ounces feta cheese, crumbled
- Choice of Protein:
- ½ cup canned lentils, drained and rinsed

or

- ½ 15-ounce can of salmon, drained

Instructions:

1. In a small bowl, whisk together the extra virgin olive oil, vinegar, dried oregano, salt, and pepper, and set aside.

2. Assemble your salad in a large mixing bowl. Combine the spring mix, chopped cucumber, olives, tomatoes, red bell pepper, and feta cheese.

3. Top with your selected choice of protein (lentils or salmon).

4. Pour the dressing from step 1 over the salad and serve.

Dinner: Veggie Kabobs
Serves 4

Ingredients:

- ¼ cup extra virgin olive oil
- 3 garlic cloves, chopped
- 1 lemon, juiced
- 1 teaspoon all-purpose seasoning (salt-free)
- sea salt and black pepper, to taste
- 2 cups mushrooms
- 1 cup cherry tomatoes
- 1 red bell pepper, chopped
- 1 green bell pepper, chopped
- 1 red onion, chopped
- 1 zucchini, chopped
- 1 yellow squash, chopped

Instructions:

1. Add olive oil, garlic, lemon juice, all-purpose seasoning, salt, and pepper to a large sealable plastic bag (like a Ziploc freezer bag).
2. Add vegetables and close the bag.
3. Shake well and place in the refrigerator for at least 1 hour. Marinating overnight is best.
4. Preheat your oven to 400 degrees Fahrenheit.
5. Slide the chopped, marinated vegetables onto the skewers.
6. Place the skewers onto a baking sheet.
7. Bake for 10 to 12 minutes until brown.

ABOUT THE AUTHOR

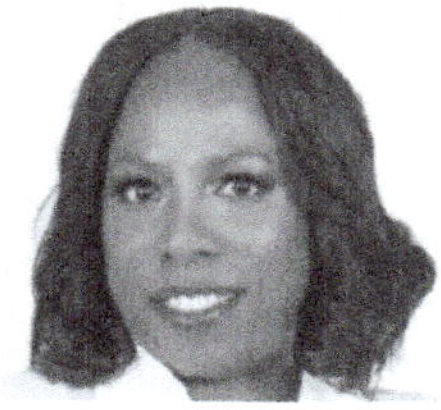

JODY DOTSON is a dedicated nutrition educator and board-certified health and wellness coach. With a personal journey of triumphing over health challenges, Jody possesses a deep understanding of the struggles faced by busy working women in their pursuit of wellness. Motivated by her own experiences, she embarked on a holistic exploration of the interconnectedness of physical and mental well-being, delving into realms such as nutrition, lifestyle medicine, and holistic health practices. This transformative odyssey inspired her to become a health coach, committed to equipping others with the tools to break free from the constraints of stress, low energy, and unfulfillment. Jody specializes in guiding women through transformations encompassing weight loss, healthier eating, and the revival of vitality, empowering them to seize control of their health and rediscover the joy in their lives. To learn more about Jody and how you can work with her visit https://jodydhealthcoach.com/

Instagram: @IamJodyDotson

Made in the USA
Monee, IL
04 November 2026

67384792R00075